CAMDEX-DS-II

Participant assessment (CAMCOG-DS-II)

A Comprehensive Assessment for Dementia in People with Down Syndrome and Others with Intellectual Disabilities
(2nd edition)

Senior editors: Jessica Beresford-Webb and Shahid H. Zaman

Sub-editors: Bessy Benejam, Rosalyn Hithersay, Frode Larsen, Sandra Loosli, Mary McCarron, Eimear McGlinchey, Silvia Sacco, Andre Strydom

Contributors: Asaad Baksh, Tonnie Coppus, Pamela Dunne, Marianne Fallon, Ségolène Falquero, Luciana Fonseca, Juan Fortea, Marianne Holland, Seán Kennelly, Johannes Levin, Ruth Mark, Diane Martet, Niamh Mulryan, Concepción Padilla, Sarah Pape, Gianluca Radic, Anne-Sophie Rebillat, Evelyn Reilly, Janette Tyrrell, Laura Videla

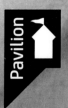

CAMDEX-DS-II Participant assessment (CAMCOG-DS-II)

Published by:

Pavilion Publishing and Media Ltd
Blue Sky Offices, 25 Cecil Pashley Way, Shoreham by Sea,
West Sussex, BN43 5FF, UK

Tel: 01273 434 943
Email: info@pavpub.com
Web: www.pavpub.com

Published 2021

ISBN: 978-1-914010-80-4

Pavilion Publishing and Media is a leading publisher of books, training materials and digital content in mental health, social care and allied fields. Pavilion and its imprints offer must-have knowledge and innovative learning solutions underpinned by sound research and professional values.

Senior editors: Jessica Beresford-Webb and Shahid H. Zaman

Sub-editors: Bessy Benejam, Rosalyn Hithersay, Frode Larsen, Sandra Loosli, Mary McCarron, Eimear McGlinchey, Silvia Sacco, Andre Strydom

Contributors: Asaad Baksh, Tonnie Coppus, Pamela Dunne, Marianne Fallon, Ségolène Falquero, Luciana Fonseca, Juan Fortea, Marianne Holland, Seán Kennelly, Johannes Levin, Ruth Mark, Diane Martet, Niamh Mulryan, Concepción Padilla, Sarah Pape, Gianluca Radic, Anne-Sophie Rebillat, Evelyn Reilly, Janette Tyrrell, Laura Videla

Publishing Editor: Ruth Chalmers, Pavilion Publishing and Media
Cover design: Emma Dawe, Pavilion Publishing and Media
Page layout and typesetting: Tony Pitt, Pavilion Publishing and Media
Printing: Ashford Press Ltd

Contents

Online material

The cancellation task stimulus 1 (p.12), the cancellation task stimulus 2 (p.13) and the circle/square/house/clock drawing page (p.18) are all available to download and print out for assessment participants from the url below.

www.pavpub.com/camdex-ds-ii

---

iv

Participant details

Name	
Address	
Reason for assessment	Clinical Research
Date of birth	
Age at assessment (years)	
Sex	Male Female

Part 1

Cognitive assessment (CAMCOG-DS-II)

Neuropsychological assessment to be conducted with the participant.

Before commencing, make sure you have the following items:

▶ CAMDEX-DS-II Picture book

▶ Pencil

▶ Wristwatch

▶ Set of keys

▶ Stopwatch

Supplementary test items:

▶ Transparent screw-top jar

▶ Small padlock with key

▶ 2 x 5p coins

▶ 2 x 10p coins

▶ 2 x 50p coins

It is important that you speak slowly and clearly. If the participant appears not to have heard or understood, repeat the question (unless the item specifically prohibits repetition).

Do not give the correct answer if a wrong answer or no answer is given.

Coding: Participants who don't know the answer, refuse to give the answer, or give a silly answer receive a score of 0 (equivalent to an incorrect answer). A score of 9 is recorded only if a question is not asked. In such cases indicate the reason for the omission of the question.

'I am going to ask you some questions now to find out about your memory and other skills. Some of them may seem very easy and others may be difficult, but we need to ask everybody the same questions.'

Orientation

188	What is your full name?	First name and surname	2
		First name (or surname) only	1
		Incorrect/failed	0
		Not asked	9
189	**What day is it today?** If no response ask: **Is it _____, _____, or _____?** (correct day of the week plus two others – correct answer 2nd)	Correct without prompt	2
		Correct with prompt	1
		Incorrect	0
		Not asked	9
190	**What month is it now?** If no response ask **Is it _____, _____, or _____?** (correct month plus the previous month and the following month – correct answer 3rd)	Correct without prompt	2
		Correct with prompt	1
		Incorrect	0
		Not asked	9
191	**What year is it now?** If no response ask: **Is it _____, _____, or _____?** (correct year plus the previous year and the following year – correct answer 2nd)	Correct without prompt	2
		Correct with prompt	1
		Incorrect	0
		Not asked	9
192	**What is the name of this place?** (if tested at home: **What is this address?**) If no response ask: **Is it _____, _____, or _____?** (correct place plus two alternatives - correct answer 2nd)	Correct without prompt	2
		Correct with prompt	1
		Incorrect	0
		Not asked	9
193	**What is the name of this town (village, city)?** If no response ask: **Is it _____, _____, or _____?** (correct town plus two alternatives – correct answer 1st)	Correct without prompt	2
		Correct with prompt	1
		Incorrect	0
		Not asked	9

Language

Comprehension

	Motor response If the participant does not complete the full sequence, the whole instruction may be repeated, without change in tone or tempo, to ensure that it has been heard and understood. Prompting and coaching stage by stage are not allowed. For questions 195–197, half marks are given for a partially correct sequence (e.g. only one of the required actions completed or actions completed in the wrong order). **I am going to ask you to do something, so please listen carefully.**		
194	**Please nod your head.**	Correct	1
		Incorrect	0
		Not asked	9
195	**Please put this pencil on your lap and then place it back on the table.**	Correct	2
		Partially correct	1
		Incorrect	0
		Not asked	9
196	**Please look at the ceiling and then look at the floor.**	Correct	2
		Partially correct	1
		Incorrect	0
		Not asked	9
197	**Please tap each shoulder twice with two fingers.**	Correct	2
		Partially correct	1
		Incorrect	0
		Not asked	9

Beresford-Webb, J & Zaman, S.(2021) *CAMDEX-DS-II Participant assessment (CAMCOG-DS-II)*

Expression

Naming

In questions 198 and 199, accurate naming is needed. Descriptions of function or approximate answers are not acceptable. Acceptable answers may depend on local usage. Errors include descriptions of function (e.g. 'used for telling time' for watch) and approximate answers (e.g. 'something you read' for book or 'light' for lamp).

In the case of approximate answers, you should say:'Can you think of another word for it?'

Tick each item correctly named and enter number correct under total.

198	Show pencil. **What is this called?** Show wristwatch. **What is this called?**	Pencil	☐
		Watch	☐
		Total	[ ]
		Not asked	9
199	**I am going to show you some pictures. Please tell me the name of each one.** Show 'pictures for naming' in picture book.	Shoe	☐
		Tree	☐
		Book	☐
		Suitcase	☐
		Clock	☐
		Lamp	☐
		Total	[ ]
		Not asked	9

Fluency

	If the participant asks for clarification, you can explain that animals include birds, insects, reptiles, etc, but only offer this explanation if you are asked for clarification. If the participant gets stuck, encourage them with: 'Can you think of any more?' Record number correct in one minute (repetitions should not be counted, but different words for variations of the same animal and specific species should be counted e.g. calf, cow, bull, fish, salmon).	
200	**I'd like you to tell me as many different animals as you can. See how many you can think of in one minute.** List all items in box.	

	Number correct	[ ]
	Recode for CAMCOG score	
	0	0
	1–4	1
	5–9	2
	10–14	3
	15+	4
	Not asked	9

Beresford-Webb, J & Zaman, S.(2021) *CAMDEX-DS-II Participant assessment (CAMCOG-DS-II)*
© Pavilion Publishing and Media Ltd 2021.

	Definitions		
201	**What do you use a hammer for?** 'Hit' gets only half marks. Some other detail should be given without prompting.	To hit (object)	2
		To hit	1
		Incorrect	0
		Not asked	9
202	**Where do people usually go to buy medicine?**	Chemist/pharmacy	1
		Incorrect	0
		Not asked	9
203	**What is a coat?** A general (abstract) definition scores 2 and a specific or limited definition scores 1.	Item of clothing	2
		Keeps you warm	1
		Incorrect	0
		Not asked	9
204	**Repetition** I am going to say something and I'd like you to repeat it after me: 'People spend money.'	Correct	2
		Partially correct	1
		Incorrect	0
		Not asked	9

Memory

New learning: Incidental memory

	Recall		
205	**I showed you some pictures a little while ago. Can you remember what they were?** Either descriptions or names are acceptable. Tick each item correctly recalled and enter number correct under total. If participant previously gave an incorrect name in question 199 but recalls it at this stage, score as correctly recalled here.	Shoe	☐
		Tree	☐
		Book	☐
		Suitcase	☐
		Clock	☐
		Lamp	☐
		Total	[ ]
		Not asked	9

	Recognition		
206	**Which one of these pictures did I show you before?** Show 'pictures for recognition' in picture book.	Shoe	☐
		Tree	☐
		Book	☐
		Suitcase	☐
		Clock	☐
		Lamp	☐
		Total	[ ]
		Not asked	9

Prospective memory

207	Show participant set of keys. **These are my keys. I'm going to put them somewhere safe.** Hide the keys (in drawer, behind curtain, etc.). Set alarm for 10 minutes. **Can you remind me about my keys when the alarm sounds?** If the alarm is going to sound while the participant is completing another question, delay the alarm until the participant completes that question.

 Beresford-Webb, J & Zaman, S.(2021) *CAMDEX-DS-II Participant assessment (CAMCOG-DS-II)*
© Pavilion Publishing and Media Ltd 2021.

Attention/concentration

	Cancellation
208	Give the participant the cancellation task stimulus 1 (p.12). (This page is available to download from www.pavpub.com/camdex-ds-ii)
	I would like you to cross out all of the images of books that you can see on this piece of paper, like this. Cross out the first image of a book. **Do this as quickly as you can and when you are finished put the pencil down on the desk.**
	Give participant a pencil, and place the cancellation task stimulus 1 on a desk.
	Ready? Go.
	After the participant finishes the task, replace the cancellation task stimulus 1 with the cancellation task stimulus 2 (p.13). (This page is available to download from www.pavpub.com/camdex-ds-ii)
	I would like you to cross out all of the images of the cars/chairs/ paintbrushes (choose one image) that you can see on this piece of paper. Do this as quickly as you can and when you are finished put the pencil down on the desk.
	Begin timing.
	Record time it takes participant to complete task (in seconds).
	If timer reaches 120 seconds, stop the task and enter 0 under total.

Record hits as number of targets crossed out.	Time	[	]
Record errors as number of incorrect targets crossed out.	Hits	[	]
Calculate [(hits – (.33 x errors)) x (60/time)] and enter under total.	Errors	[	]
	Total	[	]

Recode total into CAMCOG score		
	0	0
	1–10	1
	11–20	2
	21–30	3
	31+	4
	Not asked	9

Cancellation task – stimulus 1

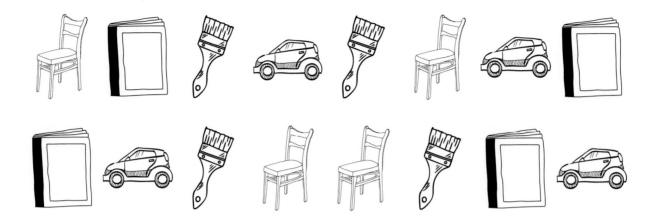

Beresford-Webb, J & Zaman, S.(2021) *CAMDEX-DS-II Participant assessment (CAMCOG-DS-II)*
© Pavilion Publishing and Media Ltd 2021.

Cancellation task – stimulus 2

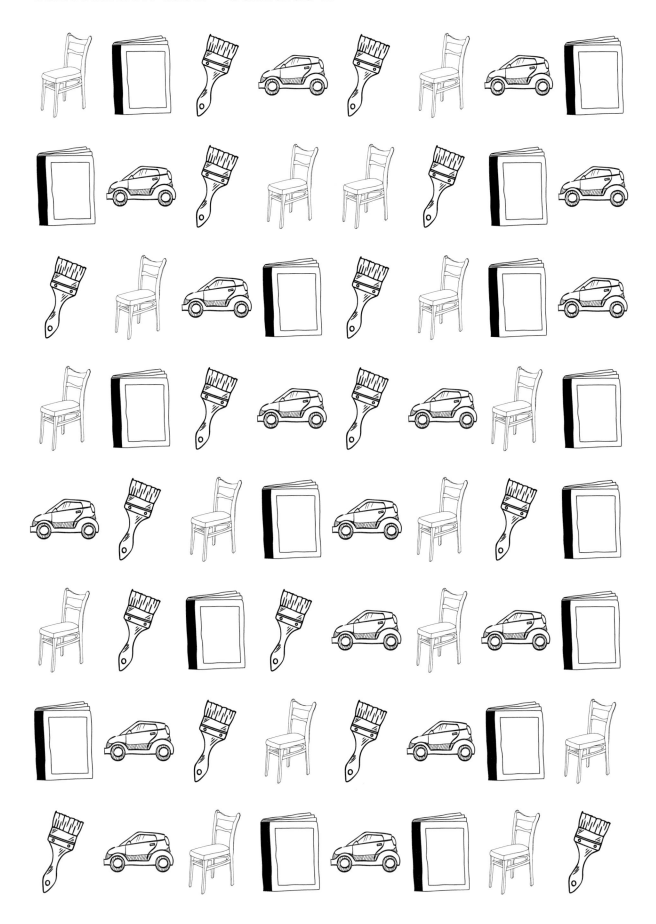

209	**Cats & dogs**

If the participant requires help with pointing, you may assist. If assistance is required, it should be introduced during the practice phase and maintained during the testing phase. Assistance with pointing should not be introduced during testing phase. Errors include both commission and omission errors.

Place the 'cats & dogs' picture from p17 of the picture book on a table directly in front of the participant. **I want you to point to and name each of the animals on this card**. Let me show you. Point to and name the first four animals.

Now you try.

If the participant gets the first four animals correct, say: '**That's it. You've got the hang of it**.' Allow the participant a maximum of three attempts.
If the participant is unable to complete the trial successfully, score as 0.

**Now I want you to point to and name all the animals on this card.
Go as quickly as you can without skipping an animal. Ready? Go.**

Begin timing. Record time taken (seconds) as T1.	T1	[ ]
Record number of uncorrected errors as E1.	E1	[ ]

Now we're going to do it differently. Every time you point to a cat, I want you to say 'dog'. Every time you point to a dog, I want you to say 'cat'. Let me show you. Name the first four animals.

Now you try.

If the participant gets the first four animals correct, say: '**That's it. You've got the hang of it**.' Allow the participant a maximum of three attempts. If the participant is unable to complete the trial successfully, score as 0.

Now try it again. Every time you point to a cat, I want you to say 'dog'. Every time you point to a dog, I want you to say 'cat'. Go as quickly as you can without skipping an animal. Ready? Go.

Begin timing. Record time taken (seconds) as T2.	T2	[ ]
Record number of uncorrected errors as E2.	E2	[ ]
Calculate (T2 – T1) and enter under time.	Time	[ ]
Calculate (E2 – E1) and enter under error.	Error	[ ]

Recode time into CAMCOG score:		Recode error into CAMCOG score:	
> 25s	0	> 3	0
16–25s	1	3–2	1
11–15s	2	1–0	2
6–10s	3	Not asked	9
< 5s	4		
Not asked	9		

Beresford-Webb, J & Zaman, S.(2021) *CAMDEX-DS-II Participant assessment (CAMCOG-DS-II)*

	Digit span		
210	I'm going to say some sets of numbers. Each time I pause, I'd like you to repeat the set back to me. Read each number string once. Tick each series correctly repeated. Discontinue after failure on both series of a given length. Score as described.	2	☐
		5	☐
		8-7	☐
		4-1	☐
		5-8-2	☐
		6-9-4	☐
		6-4-3-9	☐
		7-2-8-6	☐
		4-2-7-3-1	☐
		7-5-8-3-6	☐
		4 or 5 digit series correct	4
		3 digit series correct	3
		2 digit series correct	2
		1 digit repeated	1
		0 correct	0
		Not asked	9

Language

Comprehension

	Reading Show 'reading comprehension' in the picture book. It is not necessary for the participant to read aloud. If participant reads the instruction but fails to carry out the action, say: 'Now do what it says'. **I would like you to read this and do what it says.**		
211	'Close your eyes'	Correct	1
		Incorrect	0
		Not asked	9
212	'Give me your hand'	Correct	1
		Incorrect	0
		Not asked	9

Praxis

Copying and drawing

	The participant should draw on the sheet of paper provided (p.18). (Available to download and print from www.pavpub.com/camdex-ds-ii)		
213	**Copy this shape (circle).** A closed circular shape (circle, oval, or ellipse) is required.	Correct	1
		Partially correct	0.5
		Incorrect	0
		Not asked	9
214	**Copy this shape (square).** A closed four-sided shape (square or rectangle) is required.	Correct	1
		Partially correct	0.5
		Incorrect	0
		Not asked	9
215	**Copy this picture (3D house).** Score each component and enter number under total.		
		Outline of the house:	
		Unit correct	1
		Unit distorted, incomplete but recognisable	0.5
		Absent or unrecognisable	0
		Windows, door, and chimney in correct positions:	
		Unit correct, placed properly	2
		Unit correct, placed poorly	1
		Unit distorted, incomplete but recognisable, placed properly	1
		Unit distorted, incomplete but recognisable, placed poorly	0.5
		Absent or unrecognisable	0
		3D presentation:	
		Unit correct, placed properly	2
		Unit correct, placed poorly	1
		Unit distorted, incomplete but recognisable, placed properly	1
		Unit distorted, incomplete but recognisable, placed poorly	0.5
		Absent or unrecognisable	0
		Total	[ ]
		Not asked	9

216	**Ask the participant to draw a large clock and put all the numbers on it.** When participant has done this, say: **'Now set the hands to 10 past 11.'** Score each component and enter number under total.	

	Circular or square clockface	
	Unit correct	1
	Unit distorted, incomplete but recognisable	0.5
	Absent or unrecognisable	0

All numbers in correct position:	
All numbers present, in correct position (more or less evenly spaced within each quadrant)	2
All numbers present, not all in correct position	1
Not all numbers present, all in correct position (more or less evenly spaced within each quadrant)	1
Not all numbers present, not all in correct position	0.5
Absent or unrecognisable	0

Correct time:	
Both hands present, minute hand longer than hour hand, hour hand on 11, minute hand on 2.	2
Both hands present, one longer than the other, but one or both hands placed poorly	1
One hand present, placed properly, or two hands present, placed properly, but same size	1
One hand present, placed poorly, or two hands present, one or both poorly placed and both same size	0.5
Absent or unrecognisable	0

Total	[ ]
Not asked	9

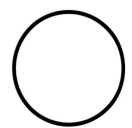

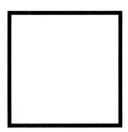

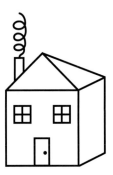

Clock:

Beresford-Webb, J & Zaman, S.(2021) *CAMDEX-DS-II Participant assessment (CAMCOG-DS-II)*
© Pavilion Publishing and Media Ltd 2021.

Memory

Registration

217	Show picture of John Brown in the picture book. **This is John Brown. Try to remember his name.** Short pause. **What is his name?** If incorrect or partially correct, say: **'His name is John Brown'.**	Correct	2
		One name only	1
		Incorrect	0
		Not asked	9
218	**I'm going to tell you where he lives. See if you can remember. He lives at 42 West Street, Bedford.** Short pause. **Where does he live?** If incorrect or partially correct, say: **'He lives at 42 West Street, Bedford'.** **Please try to remember his name and address as I will be asking you about them later on.**	Correct	2
		Partially correct	1
		Incorrect	0
		Not asked	9

Praxis

Ideomotor

	For questions 220 and 221, a correct mime is needed. If the participant uses fingers to represent knife or toothbrush, say e.g. 'Pretend you are holding a toothbrush.' Score 1 if brushing movement is made but not as though holding a toothbrush.		
219	Show me how you wave goodbye.	Correct	1
		Incorrect	0
		Not asked	9
220	Imagine you are eating with a knife. Show me how you would cut with a knife.	Correct	2
		Partially correct	1
		Incorrect	0
		Not asked	9
221	Imagine you are holding a toothbrush in your hand. Show me how you would brush your teeth with a toothbrush.	Correct	2
		Partially correct	1
		Incorrect	0
		Not asked	9

Abstract thinking

	These questions investigate the capacity to work out general relationships between objects. For questions 224 and 225, fully correct answers score 2. Partially correct answers score 1. Examples are given beside each score. If the participant says 'They are not alike', say: 'They are alike in some way. Can you tell me in which way they are alike?' **I am going to name two things and I would like you to tell me in what way they are alike. For example a dog and an elephant are alike because they are both animals.**		
222	In what way are red and yellow alike?	Colours	1
		Bright and dark	0
		Not asked	9
223	In what way are a guitar and drums alike?	Instruments	1
		Play/make music	0
		Not asked	9
224	In what way are an apple and a banana alike? For this question only, if incorrect, say: **'They are also alike because they are both kinds of fruit'**	Fruit	2
		Food, grow, have peel	1
		Round, have calories	0
		Not asked	9
	Record answer		
225	In what way are a shirt and a dress alike?	Clothing	2
		To wear, made of cloth, keep warm	1
		Have buttons	0
		Not asked	9
	Record answer		

Beresford-Webb, J & Zaman, S.(2021) *CAMDEX-DS-II Participant assessment (CAMCOG-DS-II)*

Memory

Intentional learning

226	**Recall** Show picture of John Brown in the picture book. **What was this man's name?**	Full name correct	2
		Partially correct	1
		Incorrect	0
		Not asked	9
227	**What was his address?** Tick each item recalled correctly and enter number correct under total.	42	☐
		West Street	☐
		Bedford	☐
		Total	[ ]
		Not asked	9

Visual perception

228	Show 'overlapping images' in the picture book. Point to the drawing on p.30. **Here you can see a drawing.** **This drawing is made up of five different images.** Point to the 10 images on p.31.		
	Please point to each of the images that you can see in the drawing at the left of the page. Tick each item as correct if image is recognised and enter number correct under total.	Pear	☐
		Apple	☐
		Banana	☐
		Strawberry	☐
		Cherry	☐
		Total	[ ]
		Not asked	9

Prospective memory

207	When the alarm sounds, wait for participant to remind you about your keys. If participant has not spontaneously remembered the keys, then say: **'I think I've forgotten something. Can you remember what it was?'** If there is still no response, then give this clue: **'It was my keys. Can you remember where I put them?'**		
		Item and location remembered spontaneously	3
		Item remembered with prompt	2
		Item remembered with clue	1
		Item not remembered	0
		Not asked	9

Comments

Beresford-Webb, J & Zaman, S.(2021) *CAMDEX-DS-II Participant assessment (CAMCOG-DS-II)*
© Pavilion Publishing and Media Ltd 2021.

Orientation

		Max
188 Name		(2)
189 Day		(2)
190 Month		(2)
191 Year		(2)
192 Address		(2)
193 Town		(2)
Orientation total		(12)

Language

Comprehension

		Max
194 Nod		(1)
195 Lap & table		(2)
196 Ceiling		(2)
197 Shoulder		(2)
211 Eyes		(1)
212 Hand		(1)
Total		(9)

Expression

		Max
198 Objects		(2)
199 Pictures		(6)
201 Hammer		(2)
202 Chemist		(1)
203 Coat		(2)
204 Repetition		(2)
Total		(15)

Language total		(24)

Memory

New learning

		Max
205 Recall pictures		(6)
206 Recognition		(6)
217 Register name		(2)
218 Register address		(2)
226 Recall name		(2)
227 Recall address		(3)
Memory total		(21)

Praxis

Drawing/copying

		Max
213 Circle		(1)
214 Square		(1)
215 House		(5)
216 Clock		(5)
Total		(12)

Actions to command

		Max
219 Wave		(1)
220 Knife		(2)
221 Toothbrush		(2)
Total		(5)

Praxis total		(17)

Perception

		Max
228 Overlapping images		(5)
Perception total		(5)

Executive function

Fluency

		Max
200 Animals		(4)
Total		(4)

Attention

		Max
208 Cancellation		(4)
210 Digit-span		(4)
Total		(8)

Abstract thinking

		Max
222 Colours		(1)
223 Instruments		(1)
224 Fruit		(2)
225 Clothing		(2)
Total		(6)

Prospective memory

		Max
207 Item remembered		(3)
Total		(3)

Inhibition

		Max
209 Stroop time		(4)
209 Stroop error		(2)
Total		(6)

Exec. function total		(27)

Overall total score

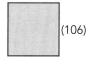

(106)

213, 214, 215 & 216 Scoring guidance

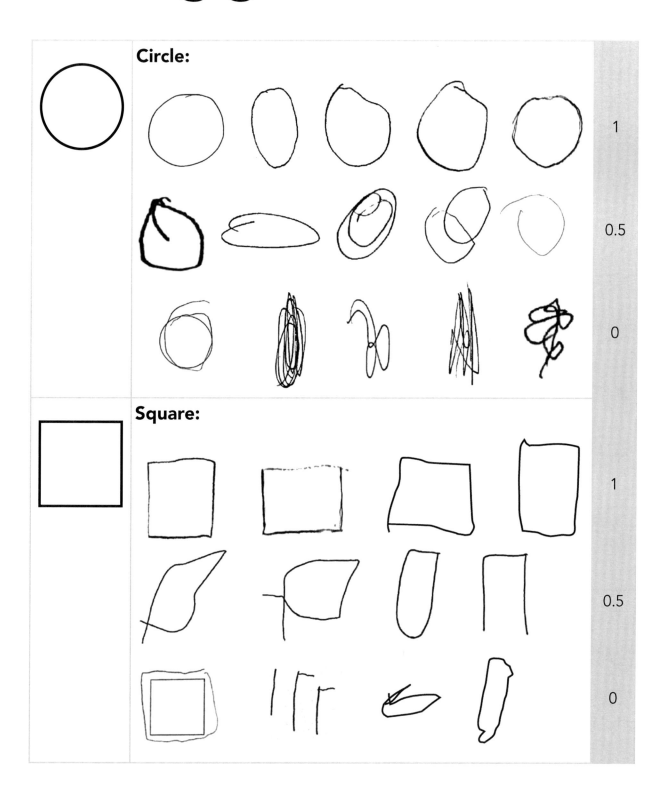

Circle:

1

0.5

0

Square:

1

0.5

0

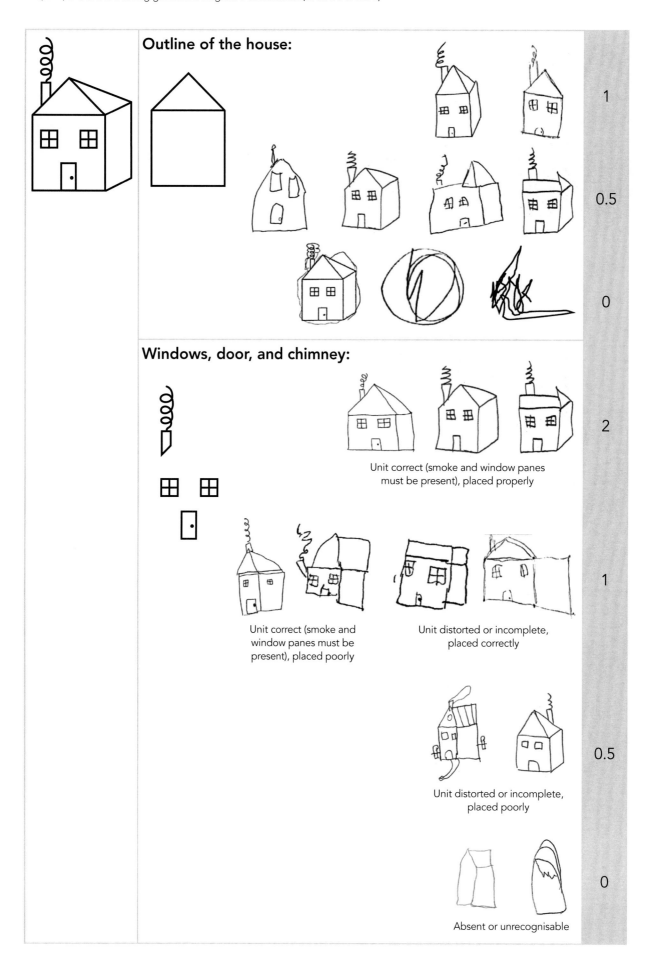

Outline of the house:

1

0.5

0

Windows, door, and chimney:

2

Unit correct (smoke and window panes must be present), placed properly

1

Unit correct (smoke and window panes must be present), placed poorly

Unit distorted or incomplete, placed correctly

0.5

Unit distorted or incomplete, placed poorly

0

Absent or unrecognisable

Beresford-Webb, J & Zaman, S.(2021) *CAMDEX-DS-II Participant assessment (CAMCOG-DS-II)*

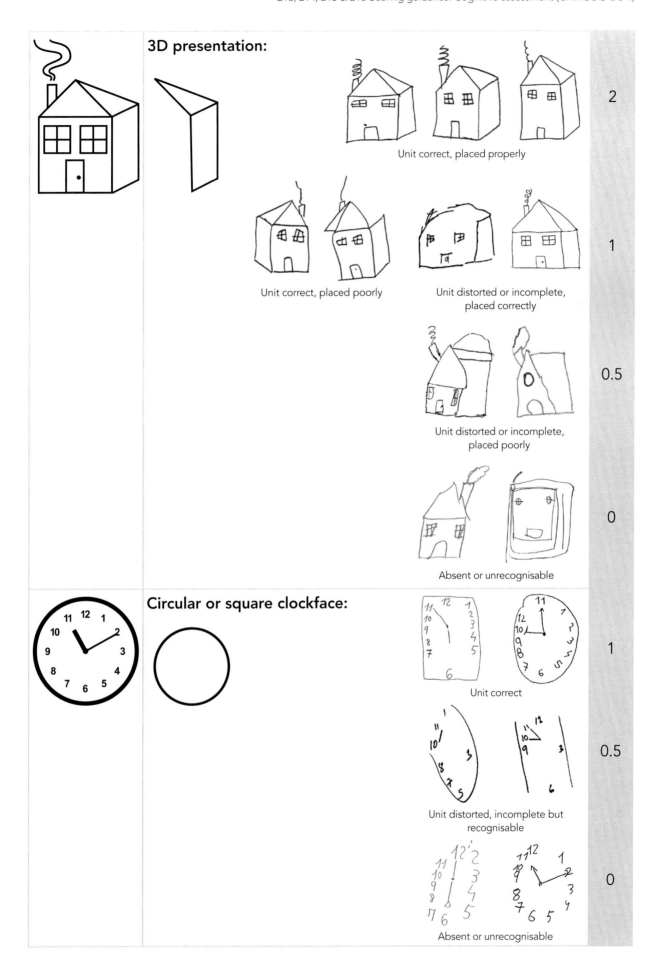

3D presentation:

Unit correct, placed properly — 2

Unit correct, placed poorly — Unit distorted or incomplete, placed correctly — 1

Unit distorted or incomplete, placed poorly — 0.5

Absent or unrecognisable — 0

Circular or square clockface:

Unit correct — 1

Unit distorted, incomplete but recognisable — 0.5

Absent or unrecognisable — 0

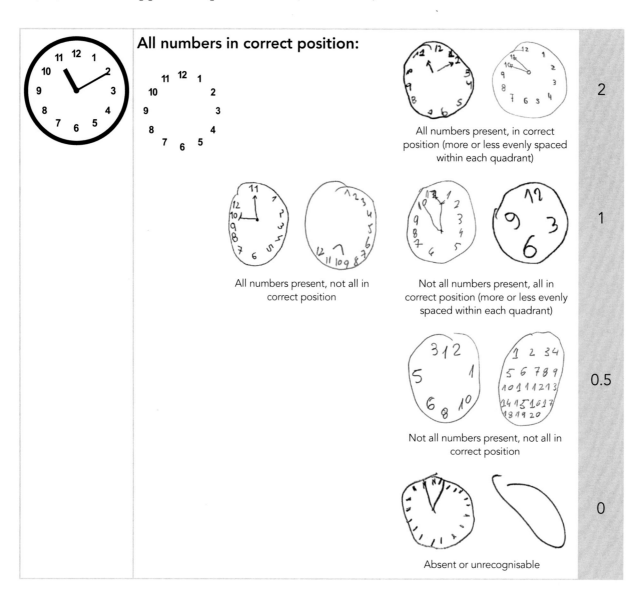

All numbers in correct position:

All numbers present, in correct position (more or less evenly spaced within each quadrant)

2

All numbers present, not all in correct position

Not all numbers present, all in correct position (more or less evenly spaced within each quadrant)

1

Not all numbers present, not all in correct position

0.5

Absent or unrecognisable

0

Beresford-Webb, J & Zaman, S.(2021) *CAMDEX-DS-II Participant assessment (CAMCOG-DS-II)*

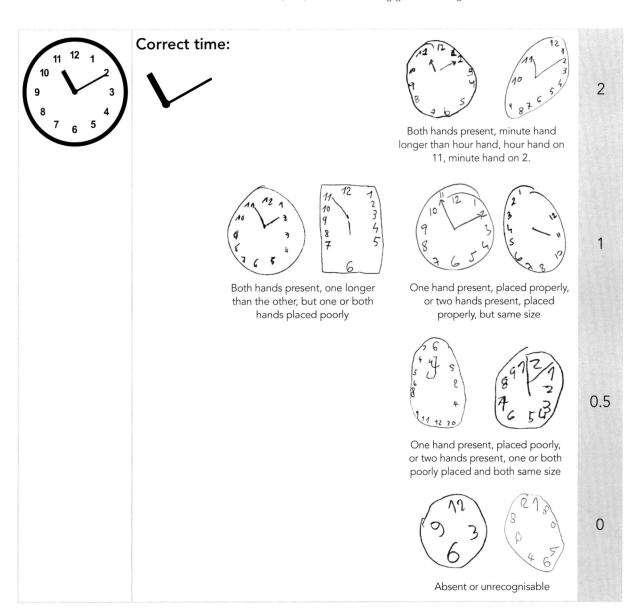

Correct time:

Both hands present, minute hand longer than hour hand, hour hand on 11, minute hand on 2.

2

Both hands present, one longer than the other, but one or both hands placed poorly

One hand present, placed properly, or two hands present, placed properly, but same size

1

One hand present, placed poorly, or two hands present, one or both poorly placed and both same size

0.5

Absent or unrecognisable

0

Supplementary test

Praxis

Refer to the 'brief praxis test scoring guidance' when scoring this task. Record the score using the 'brief praxis scoresheet'.

Read the following statements. Speak slowly and clearly.
Wait for the participant's response before moving onto the next statement.
Offer verbal approval at the end of each response, such as, 'That's good,' or 'That's fine,' or 'Good work.'

Ask the participant to stand up.

229	**Clap your hands.** Participant must bring hands together to make at least a slight sound.
230	**Lift one arm over your head.** Correct responses include lifting arm straight up in the air near head, placing hand on head, and raising hand behind head.
231	**Lift the other arm over your head.** Repeat previous item using the other arm.
232	**Turn your head to one side.** Participant's body should face forward and their head should be turned to one side.
233	**Turn your head to the other side.** Repeat previous item with head turning the opposite way.
234	**Lift one leg.** Provide access to support for the participant (e.g. table, chair, cabinet). One leg must be raised and held for two seconds. Score 4 if participant does not lean on support.
235	**Lift the other leg.** Other leg must be raised and held for two seconds. Score 4 if participant does not lean on support.

Ask the participant to sit down.

Place the small transparent jar in front of the participant and place three coins beside the jar.

| 236 | **Place each of the coins inside the jar.** If the participant switches hands during the task, instruct them not to do so and score 3. Picking coins up using thumb and fingers or sliding coins to edge of table before picking them up is acceptable. Empty the coins back on to the table and place them next to the jar. |

237	**Place each of the coins inside the jar with the other hand.** Repeat previous item using the other hand.
238	**Salute.** Hand should be raised to forehead and swung away from head.
239	**Scratch your head.** Participant should raise hand to head and use fingers to scratch back and forwards at least once.
240	**Snap your fingers.** Participant should snap middle finger against the thumb, with or without making a sound. Place a small jar with a screw cap in front of the participant.
241	**Open the jar.** Participant should unscrew the lid of the jar using both hands.
242	**Close the jar.** Participant should replace the lid of jar and screw it back on. If placed incorrectly or too loosely, prompt the participant. Place a small locked padlock and a key side by side in front of the participant.
243	**Unlock the padlock.** Key placed in keyhole and turned until the padlock opens. Allow 30 seconds before prompting. Present the padlock unlocked and open, with the key in position.
244	**Lock the padlock.** The catch should be swivelled until it snaps shut and then pressed down firmly until it is aligned with the hole. Allow 30 seconds before prompting.
245	**Point to your index/pointer finger.** Score this item as correct (4 points) or incorrect (0 points). No prompting is used. Instructions can be repeated twice. Place six coins (2 x 5p, 2 x 10p, 2 x 50p) in front of the participant in a random order. After each response, replace the coin and reshuffle.
246	**Please give me a 5-pence piece.** Score this item as correct (4 points) or incorrect (0 points). No prompting is used. Instructions can be repeated twice.
247	**Please give me a 10-pence piece.** Score this item as correct (4 points) or incorrect (0 points). No prompting is used. Instructions can be repeated twice.
248	**Please give me a 50-pence piece.** Score this item as correct (4 points) or incorrect (0 points). No prompting is used. Instructions can be repeated twice.

Beresford-Webb, J & Zaman, S.(2021) *CAMDEX-DS-II Participant assessment (CAMCOG-DS-II)*

Brief praxis test scoring guidance

4 points:	A 4-point score is given for a correct response on request without any additional verbal prompts, imitation, or modelling, or any form of physical assistance from the examiner. Four points are assigned if the participant correctly completes the item following the first or second request within 5–8 seconds.
3 points:	Providing additional verbal cues and verbal hints to the person is referred to as verbal prompting. Successful performance after the use of verbal prompts decreases the score from a maximum of 4 points (unassisted) to 3 points.
2 points:	If correct response cannot be obtained with verbal prompts, the examiner uses the next level of prompting, which is modeling. Successful performance by the participant following a modelling prompt is assigned a score of 2 points. A modelling prompt is a display by the examiner of how the correct response should be executed. Modelling is performed when the previous verbal and gestured prompts have failed to elicit the requested behaviour. The modelling is accompanied by the following verbal remarks: 'Mr/Mrs …, watch me … (e.g. make a fist, salute, etc.). Now, you do it, just like I did.'
1 point:	If modelling fails, then the examiner uses 'physical prompting'. Physical prompting is a form of 'hands-on' assistance provided by the examiner to determine whether or not the participant can perform the requested item with the addition of proprioceptive and tactile cues associated with passive movement. It is used when all other prompts have failed and it represents an attempt to make the task as easy as possible by providing the maximum number of visual and auditory cues now combined with tactile/proprioceptive as well. Three types of physical assistance are defined and used. (1) Hand over hand, in which the examiner may place their hand over the participant's hand as the participant attempts to open the lid of the jar, for example, helping the participant to turn the lid passively. (2) Moving the participant in a situation requiring standing, sitting, or walking. The examiner may place their hand under the participant's elbow to provide support in standing up or sitting down. (3) Doing something for the person. Following the physical prompt, the examiner withdraws the support given and observes whether or not the participant continues with the task to successful completion. A score of 1 point is given if the participant can perform on his/her own after physical prompting.
0 points:	Two attempts are made using physical prompting before discontinuation of the trial and assignment of a score of 0 points, meaning the subject is totally dependent on others for performing the task or is unable or unwilling to perform it.

Use the score sheet overleaf to score this task. A tick is placed in the column corresponding to the score (4, 3, 2, 1, or 0) for each item.

For items 245–248 only scores of 0 or 4 are used.

Brief praxis scoresheet

Name/ID	
Centre	
Address	
Examination date	
Examiner initials	

#	While standing	4	3	2	1	0
229	Clap your hands					
230	Lift one arm over your head					
231	Lift the other arm over your head					
232	Turn your head to the side					
233	Turn your head to the other side					
234	Lift one leg					
235	Lift the other leg					
	While seated	**4**	**3**	**2**	**1**	**0**
236	Place each of the coins in the jar					
237	. . . in the jar with the other hand					
238	Salute					
239	Scratch your head					
240	Snap your fingers					
241	Open the jar					
242	Close the jar					
243	Unlock the padlock					
244	Lock the padlock					
245	Point to your index finger					
246	Give me 5-pence piece					
247	Give me a 10-pence piece					
248	Give me a 50-pence piece					
	Total score					

4 points:

A correct response on request (one repeat allowed), without any prompts, within 5–8 seconds.

3 points:

A correct response following additional verbal cues and verbal hints.

2 points:

A correct response following a display by the examiner of how the correct response should be executed.

1 point:

A correct response following 'physical prompting' using hand over hand, in which the examiner may place their hand over the person's hand, or doing something for the person.

0 points:

Person is unable or unwilling to perform the response.

Note:

Scores of 0, 1, 2, 3, or 4 are used for items 229–244 only.
Scores of 0 or 4 only are used for items 245–248 with no prompting.

 Beresford-Webb, J & Zaman, S.(2021) *CAMDEX-DS-II Participant assessment (CAMCOG-DS-II)*
© Pavilion Publishing and Media Ltd 2021.

Part 2

Interviewer observations

To be recorded at the end of the patient/participant assessment.
Code 'yes' only if the characteristic is markedly present.

249	Self-neglect	No	Yes
250	Uncooperative behaviour	No	Yes
251	Suspiciousness	No	Yes
252	Hostility or irritability e.g. angry responses	No	Yes
253	Silly, incongruent, or bizarre behaviour	No	Yes
254	Slowness and underactivity e.g. sits abnormally still, delay in response to questions	No	Yes
255	Restlessness e.g. fidgeting, pacing, unnecessary movements	No	Yes
256	Anxiety and fear: appears frightened, worried, or somatically tense in a way that is out of proportion to the situation	No	Yes
257	Depressed mood: looks sad, mournful, or tearful; voice is low or gloomy	No	Yes
258	Lability of mood: rapidly changes from sad to happy, friendly to irritable	No	Yes
259	Flat affect: lack of spontaneous emotion or emotional response to interviewer, monotonous voice, lack of gestures	No	Yes
260	Hallucinating: behaves as though hears voices or sees visions, or admits to doing so	No	Yes
261	Speech very rapid and difficult to follow	No	Yes
262	Speech very slow with pauses between words	No	Yes
263	Speech restricted in quantity e.g. answers questions but does not say anything spontaneously	No	Yes

264	Speech rambling or incoherent, irrelevant answers to questions.	No	0	Yes	1
265	Speech slurred.	No	0	Yes	1
266	Perseveration.	No	0	Yes	1
267	Clouding of consciousness.	No	0	Yes	1
268	Speaks to self	No	0	Yes	1
269	Impaired ability to focus, sustain or shift attention.	No	0	Yes	1
270	Hypochondriacal preoccupations with somatic discomfort.	No	0	Yes	1

Beresford-Webb, J & Zaman, S.(2021) *CAMDEX-DS-II Participant assessment (CAMCOG-DS-II)*
© Pavilion Publishing and Media Ltd 2021.